Table of Contents

- RED AND YELLOW MAKE GREEN SMOOTHIE 2
- REFRESHING MINT & MELON SMOOTHIE 3
- PINA COLADA SMOOTHIE 4
- BLUE ISLAND SMOOTHIE 5
- LUCK 'O THE IRISH SMOOTHIE 6
- THINK PINK SMOOTHIE 7
- SECRET INGREDIENT SMOOTHIE 8
- ORANGE YOU GLAD YOU CAME SMOOTHIE 9
- COCONUT WATER DELIGHT SMOOTHIE 10
- DREAMY CRANBERRY SMOOTHIE..................................11
- GOOD FOR YOUR HEART SMOOTHIE 12
- MEAN AND GREEN SMOOTHIE 13
- STRAWBERRY DELIGHT SMOOTHIE 14
- SESAME MANGO SMOOTHIE 15
- FEELING BLUE SMOOTHIE 16
- GREEN COLADA SMOOTHIE...17
- LEAN AND GREEN SMOOTHIE 18
- CHICORY AND PRUNE SMOOTHIE 19
- PINEAPPLE, STRAWBERRY AND COCONUT SMOOTHIE 20
- BERRY PINEAPPLE-RITA SMOOTHIE 21
- CREAMY MANGO SMOOTHIE 22
- SIMPLE STRAWBERRY BANANA SMOOTHIE 23
- MANGO ARUGULA SMOOTHIE 24
- KREAMY KALE SMOOTHIE...25
- CHOCOLATE LOVER'S SMOOTHIE 26

RED AND YELLOW MAKE GREEN SMOOTHIE

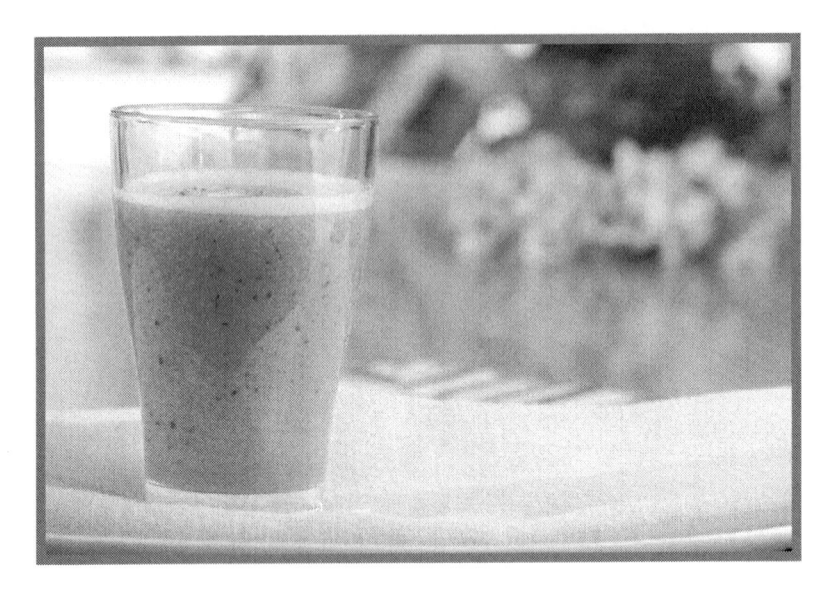

This smoothie packs quite a punch when you add the high fiber content of raspberries with the nutrient dense kale. You'll get vitamin-C from the berries and pineapples along with iron, calcium and vitamin-K from the kale. This smoothie would be great to down in the morning or if you are feeling a bit under the weather.

Yields: 1-2 servings

Ingredients:
1 cup freshly cut pineapple chunks
½ cup raspberries
1-2 leaves of kale (any kind of kale will work)
½ English cucumber, peeled and roughly chopped
Ice
Water

Method:
1. Place a small amount of water and ice cubes in blender.
2. Place remaining ingredients in blender and blend until smooth.

REFRESHING MINT & MELON SMOOTHIE

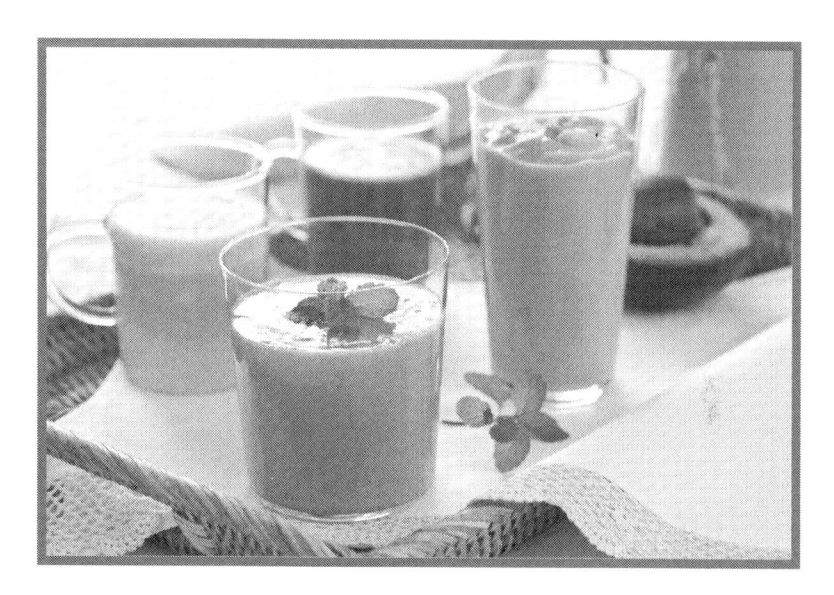

Honeydew is one of the last popular melons but works great in smoothies as it adds density and a mild flavor that's not too overpowering. Combined with mint, this smoothie seems perfect for a warm summer's evening. Besides adding a refreshing, light taste to smoothies, mint is high in Vitamin-A, a nutrient essential for healthy vision.

Yields: 2 servings

Ingredients:
2 cups chopped honeydew
1 cup chopped English cucumber
12 mint leaves picked removed from the stems
2-4 tablespoons fresh limejuice, to taste
1 teaspoon raw honey

Method:
Place all of the ingredients in a blender and blend until smooth.

Serves 2

PINA COLADA SMOOTHIE

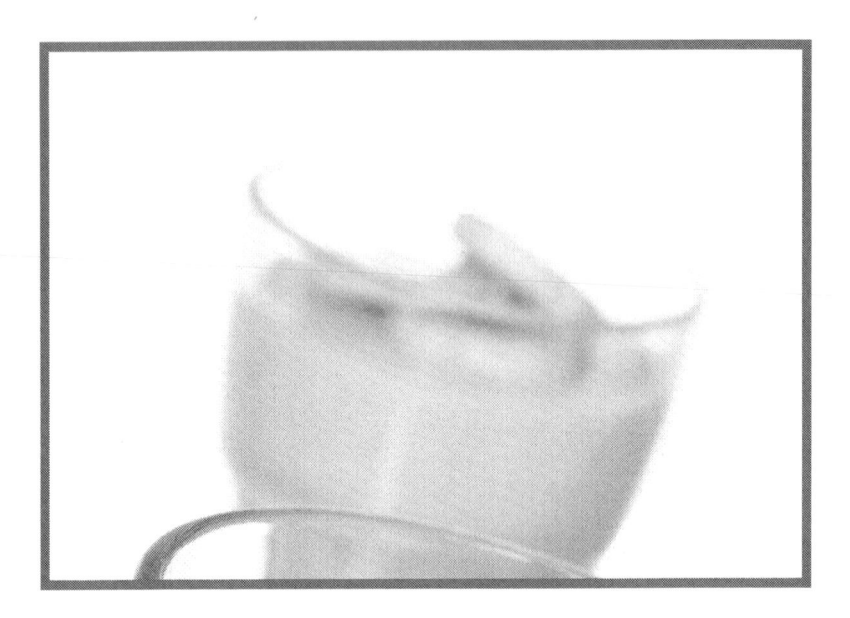

While your traditional pina colada is milky white, this smoothie will be dark green in color thanks to the collard greens. If you prefer to work with the actual coconut as opposed to the coconut milk, go ahead! Just be sure to choose a young coconut with soft, creamy flesh that can be scooped out. If using canned coconut milk, make sure it is unsweetened.

Yields: 3-4 servings

Ingredients:
13.5-oz can of unsweetened coconut milk

Banana

16-ounce bag frozen pineapple
1/2 bunch of collard greens, stems removed (4-5 large leaves)

Method:

1. Pour the coconut milk into the blender.
2. Add remaining ingredients and blend until smooth.

BLUE ISLAND SMOOTHIE

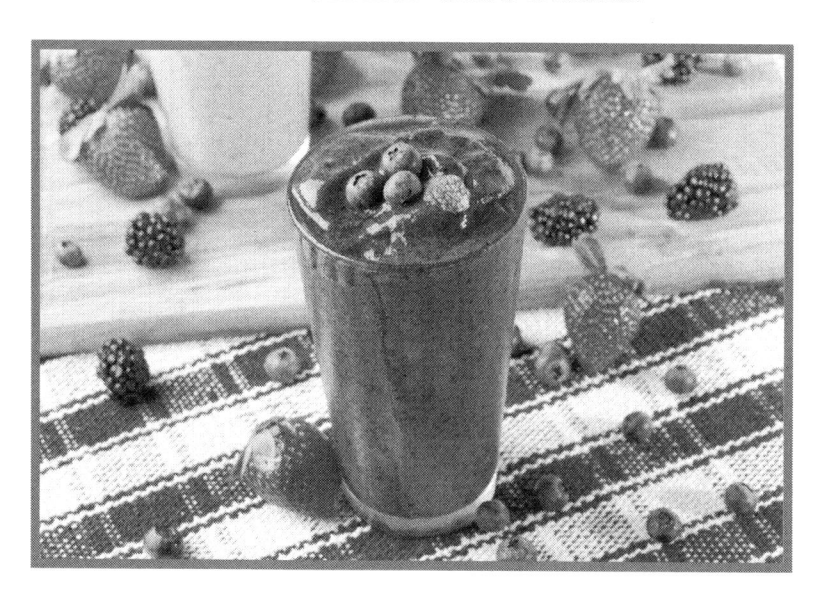

Whether you are in the middle of winter and longing to be sitting cool beverages on white beaches or melting in the heat of summer, this smoothie is always a winner! If you want to add a crunchy texture, opt for frozen blueberries and frozen pineapple. If it comes out a little too sweet for your taste then you can always half the orange juice and add water. Kick off your shoes, relax and imagine ocean waves lulling you to sleep as you sip this tropical smoothie!

Yields: 2 servings

Ingredients:
1 cup fresh blueberries
1 banana
½ cup chopped fresh pineapple
½ cup orange juice

Method:
1. Add all ingredients to blender and blend.
2. If smoothie is too thick, add a bit more orange juice to thin it out.

LUCK 'O THE IRISH SMOOTHIE

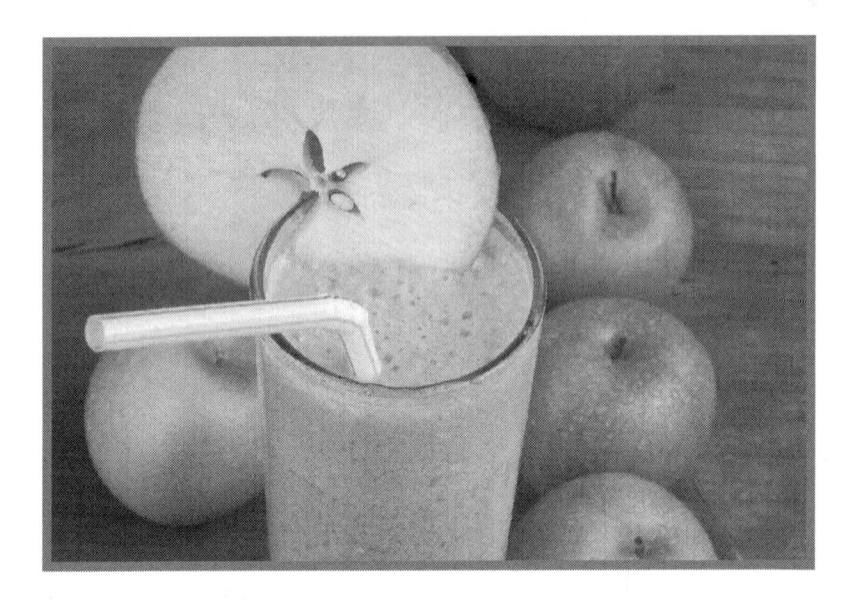

What St. Patrick's Day (or any day for that matter?) isn't perfect without a green smoothie to start your day? The spinach will keep this smoothie nice and dark while adding fiber and cancer fighting flavonoids to your diet. The fruit will keep the smoothie nice and sweet making this a perfect combination of bitter and sweet. Enjoy sipping this shamrock smoothie (much healthier than the milkshake variety)!

Yields: 3 servings

Ingredients:
2 bananas, peeled
½ cup frozen peaches
1 medium apple, cored and cut into wedges
2 handfuls fresh spinach leaves
1/3 cup water, plus more as needed

Method:
1. Place the water in the blender before adding all other ingredients. Puree into smooth and creamy.
2. Add additional water as needed if smoothie is too thick.

THINK PINK SMOOTHIE

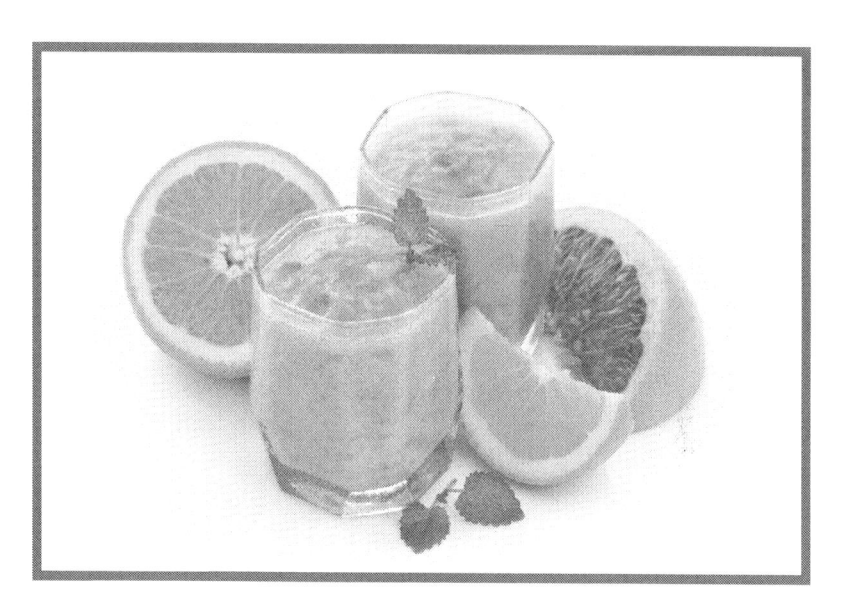

It's rare to find grapefruits in smoothies, which is why this recipe gets a five-star rating when it comes to skin protection and fighting cholesterol. Since grapefruit is low in calories, you are getting a powerhouse of nutrients without the high calorie content of some fruits. If you have a hard time with ginger then you can add a bit of honey instead. If the smoothie is still too bitter, try halving the water with fruit juice.

Yields: 1 serving

Ingredients:
1 ruby red grapefruit, peeled, seeded, and chopped
2 cups fresh or frozen strawberries, stems removed
1 sweet apple (such as Honeycrisp or Pink Lady), cored and chopped
1 inch fresh ginger, peeled and chopped
1 cup water

Method:
1. Place the water in the blender and then add all other ingredients. Blend until smooth.
2. Add additional water as needed if smoothie is too thick.

SECRET INGREDIENT SMOOTHIE

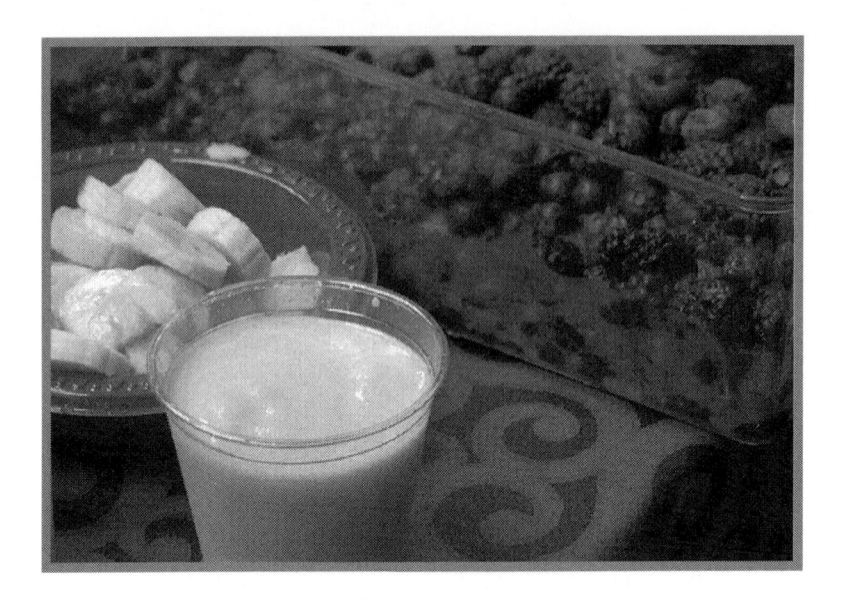

Although greens are popular in smoothies, too many people are put off by the putrid color they can leave behind. This smoothie is great because it packs the nutrient power of spinach without the grotesque color which means you can trick just about anyone into drinking it! If you want a crunchy flavor without the ice, use frozen raspberries and bananas.

Yields: 2 servings

Ingredients:
1 medium orange, peeled and seeded
1 medium banana
2 cups raspberries
2 cups packed baby spinach
5 dried dates, pitted
2 tablespoons ground flaxseeds (optional)
1 cup ice, if using fresh berries

Method:
1. Roughly chop the orange, banana, spinach, and dates.
2. Pour water into blender and add chopped fruits and vegetables. Blend until smooth, adding a little water to thin out if necessary.

ORANGE YOU GLAD YOU CAME SMOOTHIE

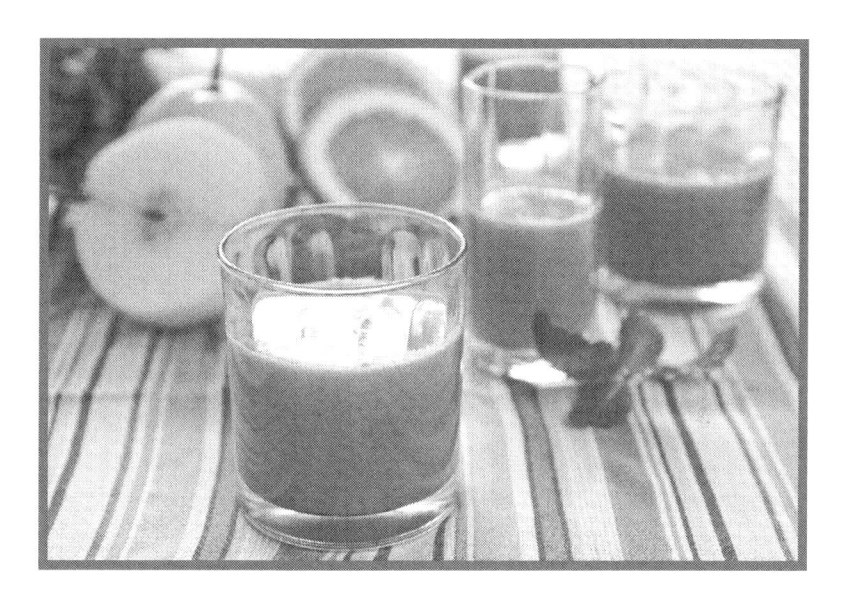

If you are used to having orange juice with your breakfast, this smoothie is a perfect way to start your day! The mango and carrot juice will bring the familiarity of your morning beverage along with an unbelievable amount of beta-carotene. If you don't have a fancy juicer to make your carrot juice, simply add 2 lbs of carrots and a small amount of water to blender. Blend until finely pureed. Pour the carrots into a pitcher along with 2 cups of hot water and let it soak for 30 minutes. Strain the juice and the liquid is ready to add to your smoothie.

Yields: 2 servings

Ingredients:
1 mango, seeded and chopped (or 1 ½ cups frozen mango chunks)
1 cup fresh carrot juice
Dash freshly grated nutmeg
½ cup ice cubes (ignore if using frozen mango)

Method:
Place all ingredients in blender and puree until smooth.

COCONUT WATER DELIGHT SMOOTHIE

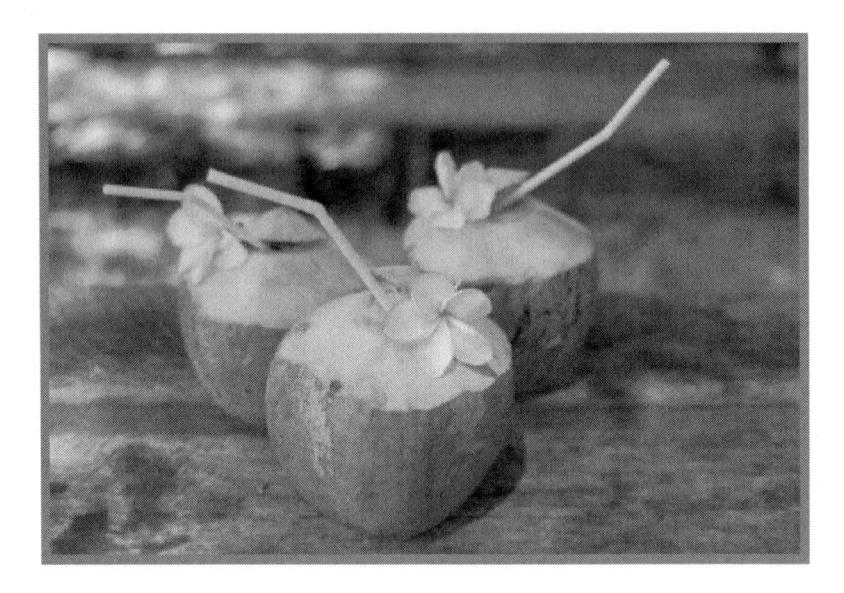

Coconut water used to be hard to come by but now, thanks to its growing popularity, you can find it at almost any convenience or grocery store. Just make sure it is unsweetened with no added flavorings. If you'd rather have a denser smoothie, you can easily substitute more coconut milk.

Yields: 4 servings

Ingredients:
½ lb. strawberries (fresh or frozen)
3 large ripe bananas, peeled
1 cup unsweetened coconut water
¼ cup coconut milk
Raw honey, to taste

Method:
1. If using fresh strawberries, wash and remove stems.
2. Combine all ingredients except honey in blender.
3. Blend until smooth, adding honey to taste.

DREAMY CRANBERRY SMOOTHIE

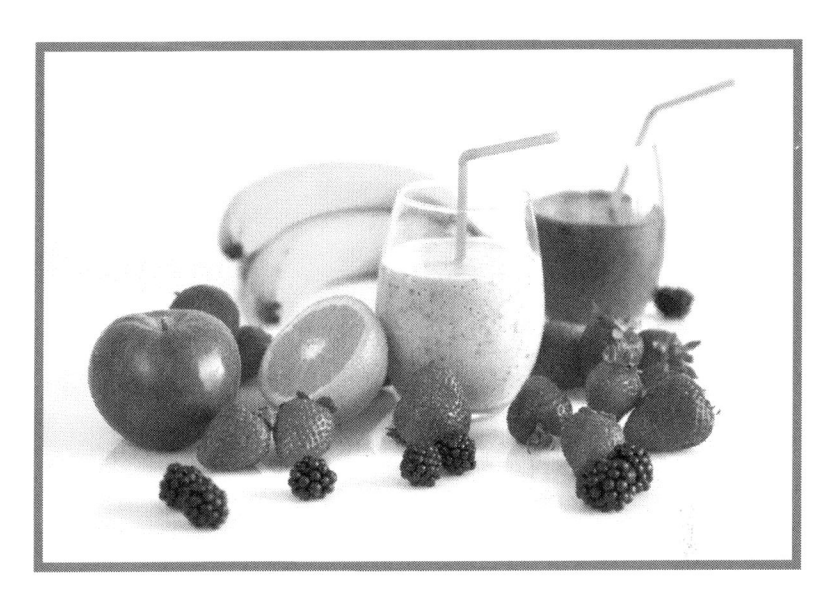

If you think cranberries are only for Thanksgiving, think again! These little berries are loaded with vitamin-C as well as high in dietary fiber. Cranberries are popular among women as they can fight off urinary tract infections and aid in digestive health. Since this smoothie does seem to have a festive list of ingredients, it's perfect for the holidays or on snowy Christmas mornings when you don't feel like cooking up a huge breakfast.

Yields: 2 servings

Ingredients:
½ cup frozen cranberries
1 medium frozen banana, peeled and sliced
2 Clementine oranges, peeled and seeded
2 Medjool dates, pitted (or substitute 2 tablespoons honey)
½ cup cranberry juice (or water)
¼ teaspoon pure vanilla extract
¼ teaspoon ground cinnamon
½ cup ice
Splash of sparkling water, optional

Method:
1. Combine all ingredients in a blender and blend until smooth.
2. If desired, mix a good splash of sparkling water when serving.

GOOD FOR YOUR HEART SMOOTHIE

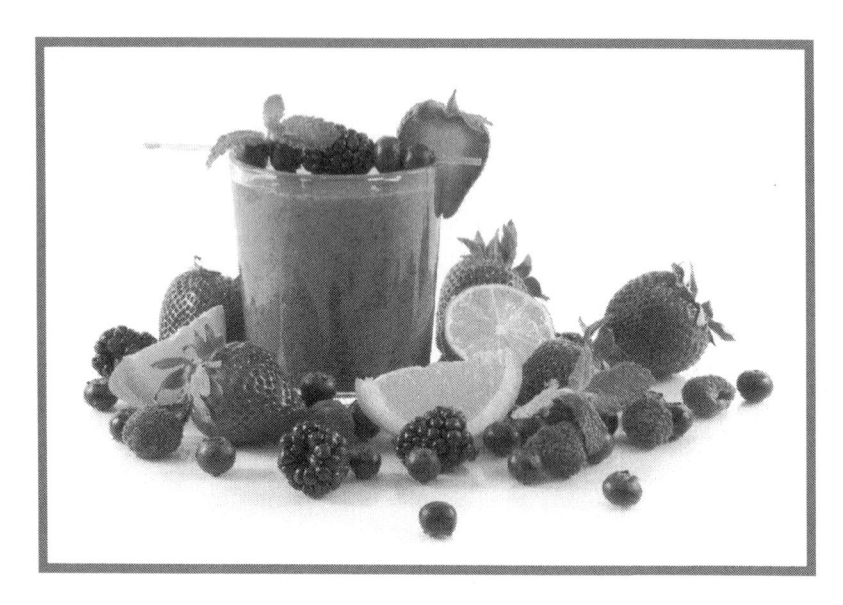

This super simple recipe is perfect when you are in a hurry or if you are craving a light, sweet snack. Loaded with pomegranate juice to give you a healthy dose of antioxidants, this is a powerhouse smoothie perfect for anytime of the day or night. Male or female, young or old, the berries and pomegranate juices are high in folic acid and will load you up with vitamin-C to stave off any unwanted colds.

Yields: 2 servings

Ingredients:
2 cups mixed frozen berries, fresh or frozen
1 cup unsweetened pomegranate juice
1 cup water

Method:
Combine all ingredients in a blender and blend until smooth.

MEAN AND GREEN SMOOTHIE

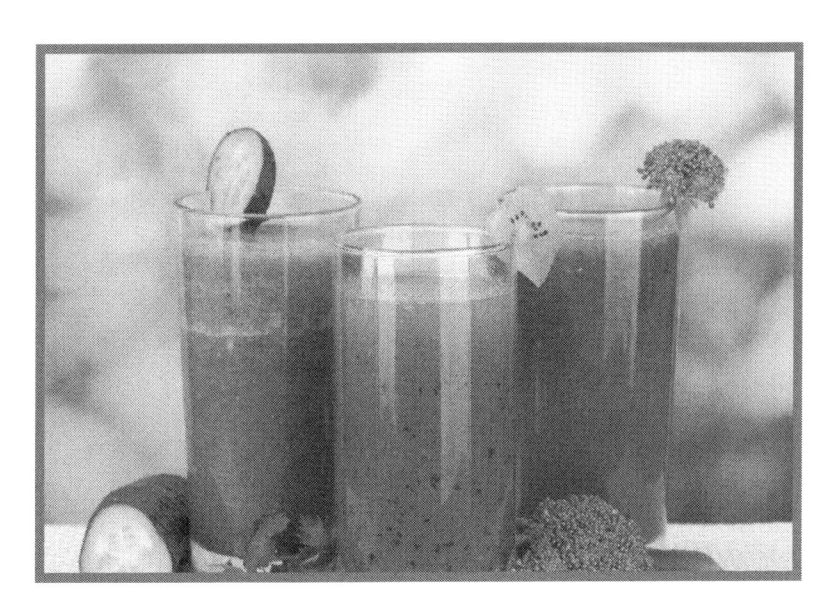

You'll probably be surprised at the sweetness of this smoothie considering there's only one banana but it masques the taste of the spinach and delivers a refreshing, frothy breakfast treat. The almond milk gives this a silky texture and the flaxseed adds a healthy amount of omega-3 essential fatty acids. If you're brave enough to give it a try, it will undoubtedly become part of your healthy morning, afternoon or evening routine!

Yields: 1 serving

Ingredients:
1 cup unsweetened almond milk
2 large handfuls of spinach
1 tablespoon ground flaxseed
3-4 ice cubes
1 banana

Method:
1. Pour almond milk into the blender and then add all other ingredients.
2. Blend until smooth.

STRAWBERRY DELIGHT SMOOTHIE

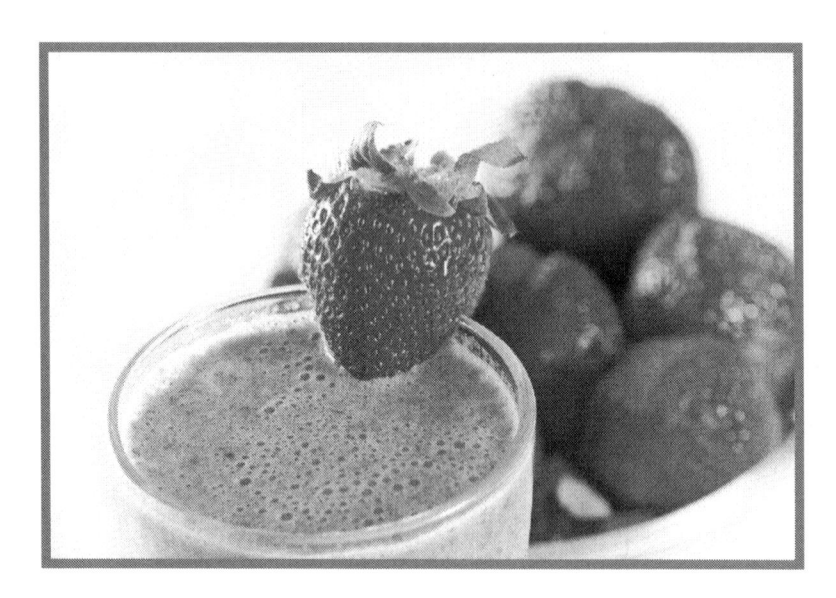

It's been in recent decades that Kefir made its way into American grocery stores but it has been a staple in Eastern Europe since the 1800's. Packed with healthy bacteria known as probiotics, Kefir is a delicious way to aide digestion and make sure your immune system is functioning nice and strong. Lifeway recently came out with a frozen variety that makes this smoothie delicious enough to be a dessert!

Yields: 2 servings

Ingredients:
1 cup strawberry frozen Kefir
1 cup fresh strawberries
1/2 cup almond milk
3-4 ice cubes

Method:
1. Remove all stems from the strawberries.
2. Combine all ingredients in a blender and blend until smooth.

SESAME MANGO SMOOTHIE

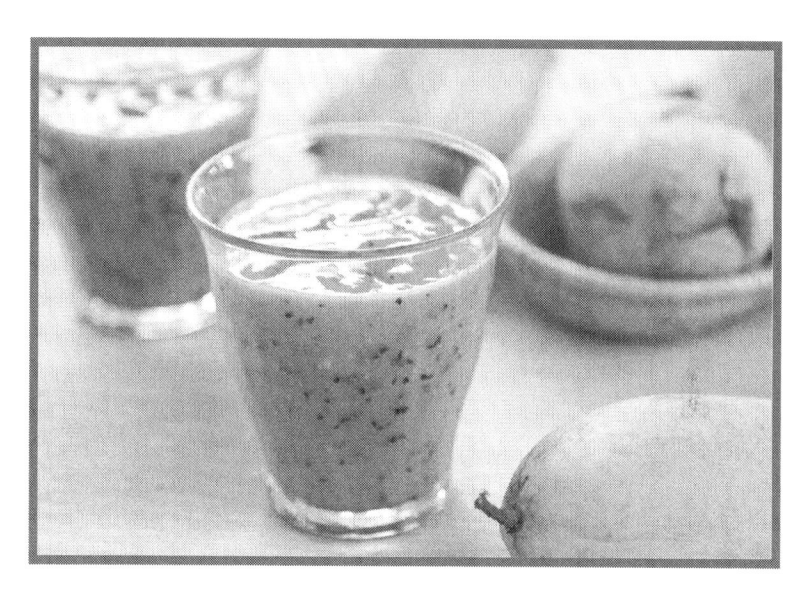

Tahini probably isn't a staple in most people's pantries. It's a thick paste made from ground up sesame seeds and usually comes in a tube or jar. If you've ever tasted the earthy, gritty texture of hummus, then you've unknowingly consumed tahini. It contains a variety of vitamin-B's and is also a good source of calcium. If you are not used to the taste of sesame, it might be a bit overpowering at first so feel free to adjust the amount used until your taste buds have acclimated.

Yields: 1 serving

Ingredients:
1 cup slightly thawed frozen mango
1 Tbsp tahini
1 Tbsp limejuice
½ cup water

Method:
Blend all ingredients until smooth.

FEELING BLUE SMOOTHIE

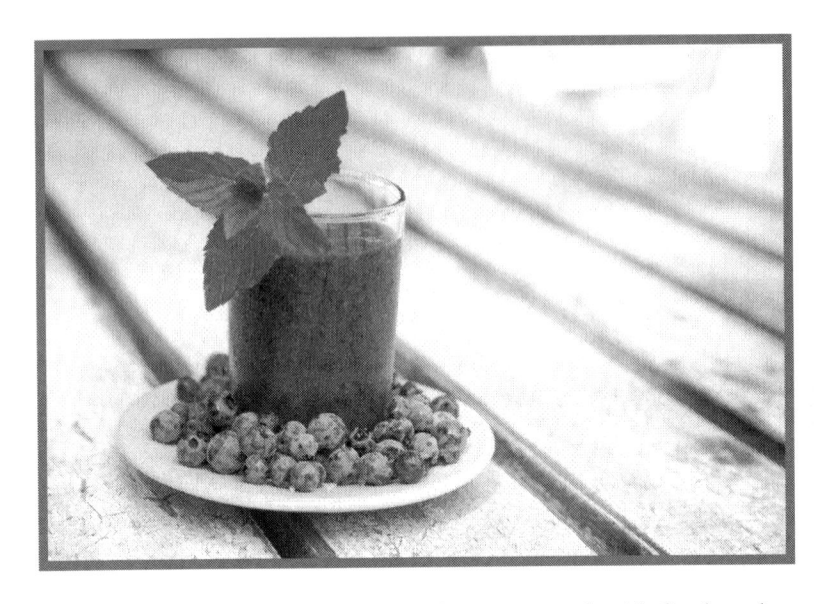

Since the word 'antioxidant' is the new catch phrase among health food marketers, don't be fooled into buying expensive pills and juices when you can easily pop a few blueberries! More than any other fresh fruit, these little berries have the highest antioxidant capacity. Combine that with the healthy fat and high vitamin content found in avocados, and this smoothie is a guaranteed pick-me-up on those days when your feet are dragging and your late-night TV habit is catching up with you!

Yields: 1 serving

Ingredients:
1 cup frozen blueberries
½ ripe avocado
¼ cup orange juice
½ cup fresh mint leaves
1 tsp fresh lemon juice
½ cup water

Method:
Place all ingredients in blender and blend until smooth.

GREEN COLADA SMOOTHIE

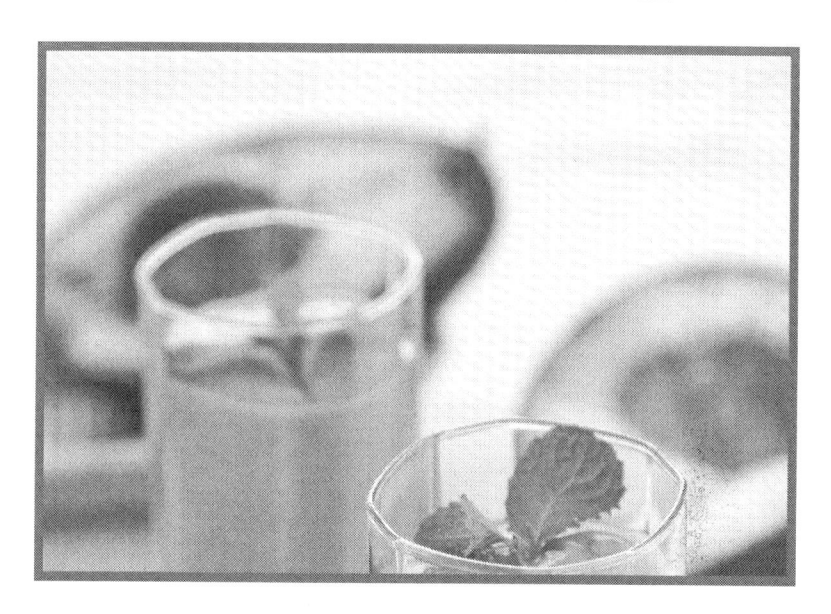

This recipe combines some of the basic fruits found in your classic smoothie: pineapples and bananas. Throw in an avocado for a little kick of healthy fats and vitamins, and you've got a new take on a classic island treat. Hang a little umbrella over the side and sprinkle some coconut flakes on top while imagining yourself lounging on a Caribbean beach soaking up the rays! If you don't have coconut milk on hand almond milk is a good substitution.

Yields: 1 serving

Ingredients:
½ cup orange juice
½ cup frozen pineapple
½ avocado
½ of a frozen banana
 tsp limejuice
 Tbsp unsweetened coconut milk
Pinch of sea salt

Method:
Place all ingredients in blender and blend until smooth.

LEAN AND GREEN SMOOTHIE

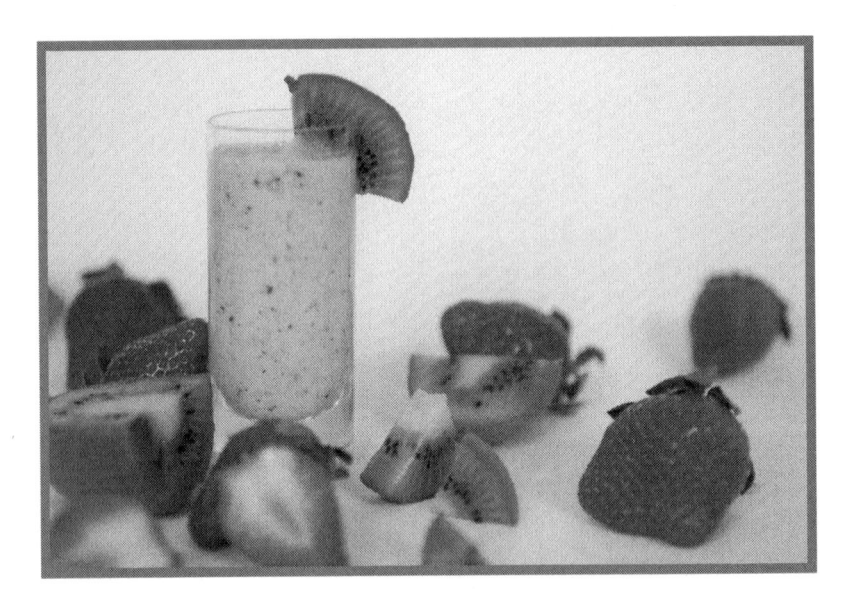

While some fruits show up in smoothies all the time, kiwi is the often-neglected ingredient. There's a reason why this shows up in natural skincare products, as it is high in Vitamin E and Vitamin C, which helps maintain collagen for firm, younger looking skin. When picking your honeydew to add to the smoothie, look for a creamy white rind and a firm light green middle. Overripe honeydew has a lower nutritional content that, while still beneficial, won't pack quite the nutritional punch.

Yields: 2 servings

Ingredients:
2 cups cubed, peeled seeded honeydew melon
2 cups crushed ice
1 ¼ cups peeled, cubed kiwi
10 large fresh mint leaves
1 tablespoon fresh limejuice
1 tablespoon raw honey

Method:
Place all ingredients in blender and blend until smooth.

CHICORY AND PRUNE SMOOTHIE

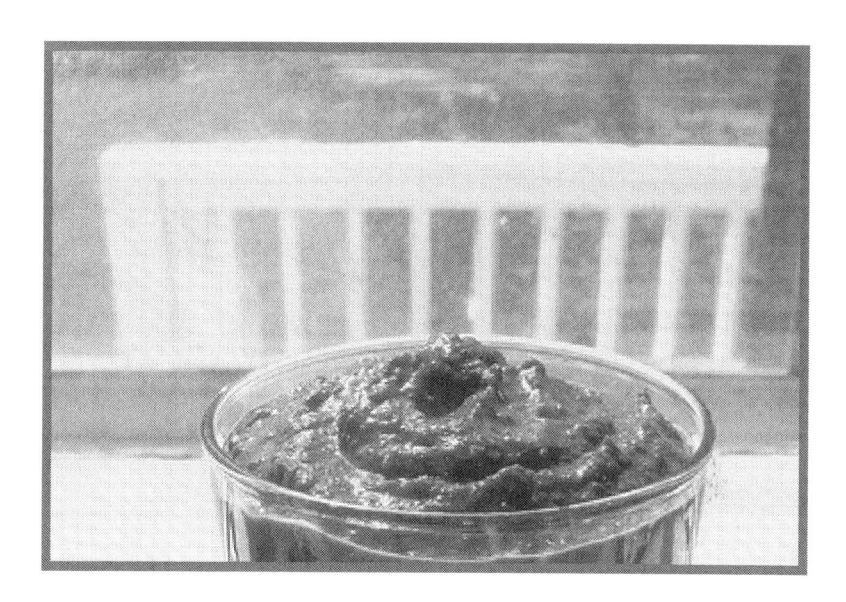

This smoothie is packed with digestive power and is perfect if you are, let's just say, a little irregular! You should be able to find chicory root instant coffee at just about any health food or you could always order online. If you are trying to kick the habit of traditional morning coffee, this smoothie is great because it still offers a rich creamy coffee-like taste without all of the acid and caffeine.

Yields: 2 servings

Ingredients:
1 cup boiling water
2 tsp chicory root instant coffee substitute (TRY: Pero Instant Natural Beverage)
3 pitted, unsweetened prunes
1 cup unsweetened almond milk
2 tsp unsweetened almond butter
5 ice cubes

Method:
1. In a small saucepan, combine chicory, prunes and boiling water. Let soak for 10 minutes.
2. Transfer mixture and all liquid to a blender. Add remaining ingredients and blend.

PINEAPPLE, STRAWBERRY AND COCONUT SMOOTHIE

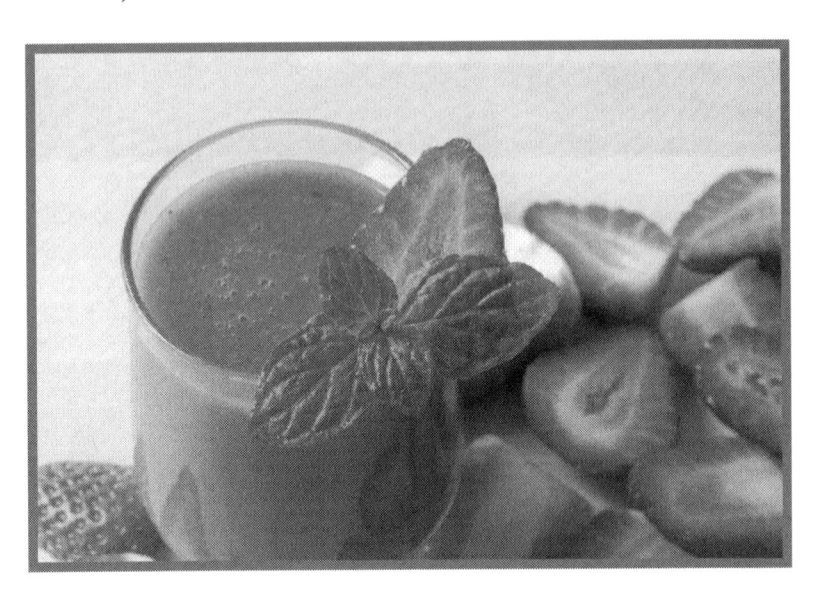

This smoothie is about as fruity as it gets since there's nothing green hidden in the mix of ingredients. Perfect for a refreshment on a hot summer day or to add some healthy medium-chain triglycerides (MCTs) from all of the coconut oil to your diet. This is also a great way to get your children to digest coconut milk as the pineapples and strawberries will entice people of all ages to drink up!

Yields: 2-3 servings

Ingredients:
1 cup coconut milk
2 teaspoons coconut oil
8 ounces frozen pineapple chunks
6 ounces frozen strawberries

Method:
1. Add coconut milk to your blender following by remaining ingredients.
2. Blend until smooth and creamy.

BERRY PINEAPPLE-RITA SMOOTHIE

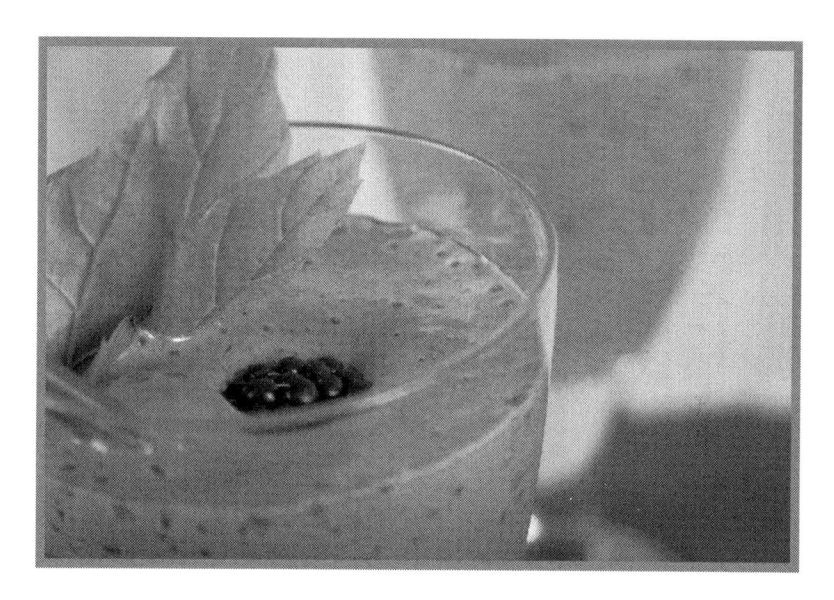

Everything about this smoothie screams backyard barbeque especially since it offers your guests a margarita type beverage without the alcohol. If you are looking for a fun garnish, try skewering a few of the blueberries on a toothpick or sticking a couple of fresh pineapples on the rim. There's also nothing that says you have to reserve this recipe for hot summer days. Why not sip a little berry pineapple-rita smoothie while soaking in a hot tub after a long day at work?

Yields: 1 serving

Ingredients:
8 oz fresh, frozen blueberries
4 fl oz pineapple juice
. tsp raw honey
. large watermelon wedge, peeled, seeded and cubed
Bar salt (optional)

Method:
1. Dip the rim of your smoothie glass in water and then in bar salt.
2. Place remaining ingredients in blender and blend until smooth.

CREAMY MANGO SMOOTHIE

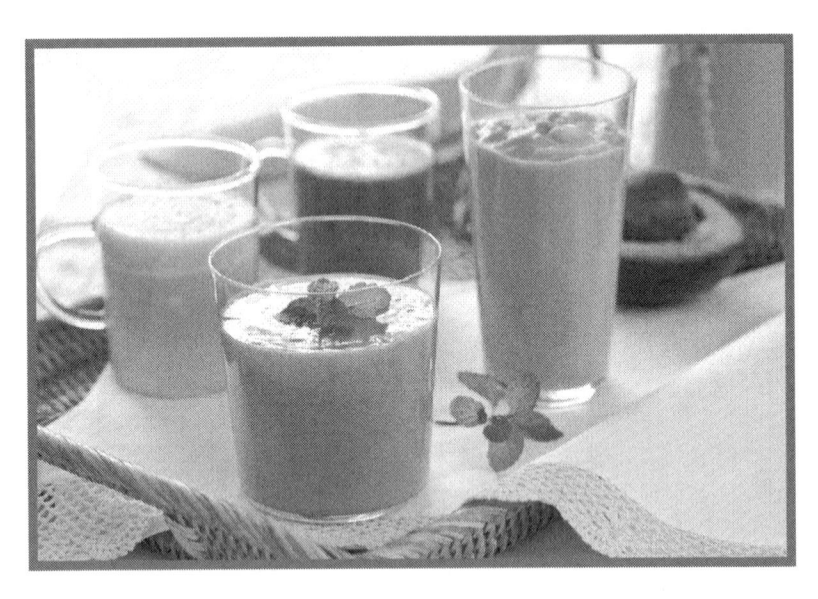

Similar to an orange Julius smoothie, this recipe simply swaps out the orange for mango and adds a much healthier dairy alternative in the almond milk. Small, manila mangoes will add to the sweet, creamy texture and are really the best type for this smoothie. If you have to choose the more traditional Tommy Atkins variety of mango, accept the fact it will add a more tart flavor.

Yields: 4 servings

Ingredients:
1 ½ cups diced ripe mango
1 cup ice cubes
1 pinch salt
½ teaspoon fresh lemon juice
1 ½ cups unsweetened almond milk

Method:
Place all ingredients in blender and blend until smooth.

SIMPLE STRAWBERRY BANANA SMOOTHIE

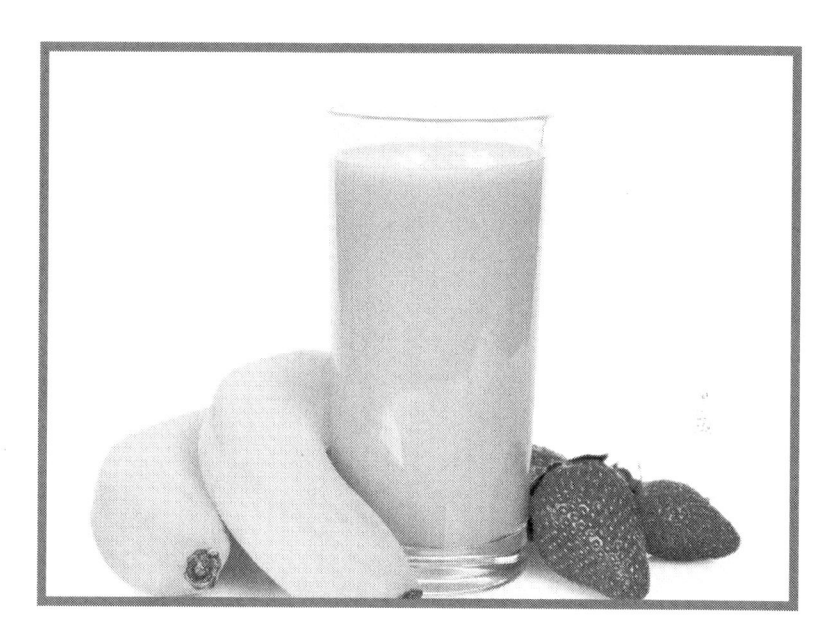

This is about as traditional as it gets when it comes to smoothie making. It combines two fruits that you can find year round: frozen strawberries and bananas. This smoothie is great in the morning or as an afternoon snack when you need a little pick me up after a long day's work. Because it contains orange juice and honey it might be on the sweeter side. If you find you don't need all the sweetness, feel free to adjust the amounts.

Yields: 2 servings

Ingredients:
2 cups frozen strawberries
2 bananas
1½ cups unsweetened almond milk
1 cup orange juice
1 tablespoon raw honey

Method:
Place all ingredients in blender and blend until smooth.

MANGO ARUGULA SMOOTHIE

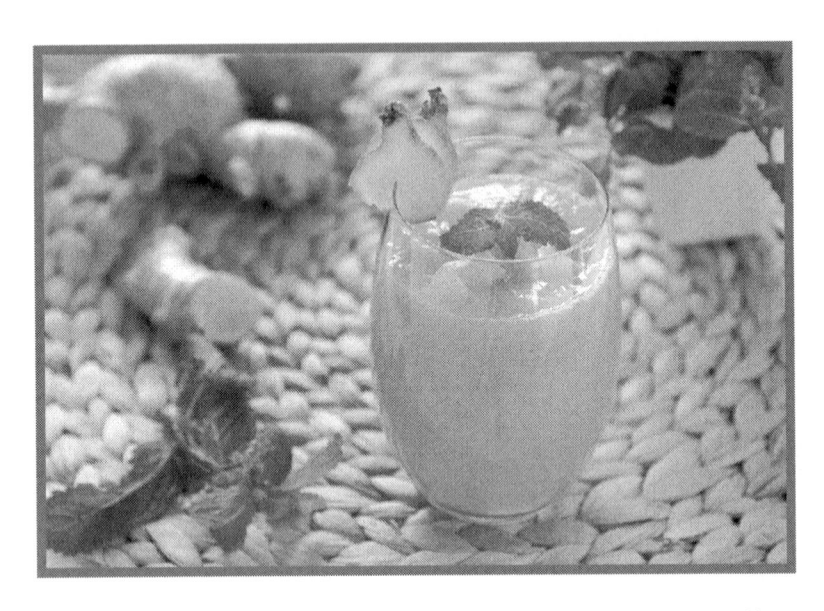

Because arugula is more often associated with salads, it might take some effort to drop the leaves into your blender for a smoothie. You don't want to swap them out or substitute because you'll be missing out on calcium, vitamins A, C and K, not to mention iron. Since arugula is best consumed raw, this makes for a perfect smoothie combination.

Yields: 2 servings

Ingredients:
3 ounces arugula
1 ripe mango, peeled and pitted
1 lemon, peeled (remove white pith, too) and seeded
1 teaspoon minced or grated fresh ginger
1 cup water
½ cup ice

Method:
Place all ingredients in blender and blend until smooth.

KREAMY KALE SMOOTHIE

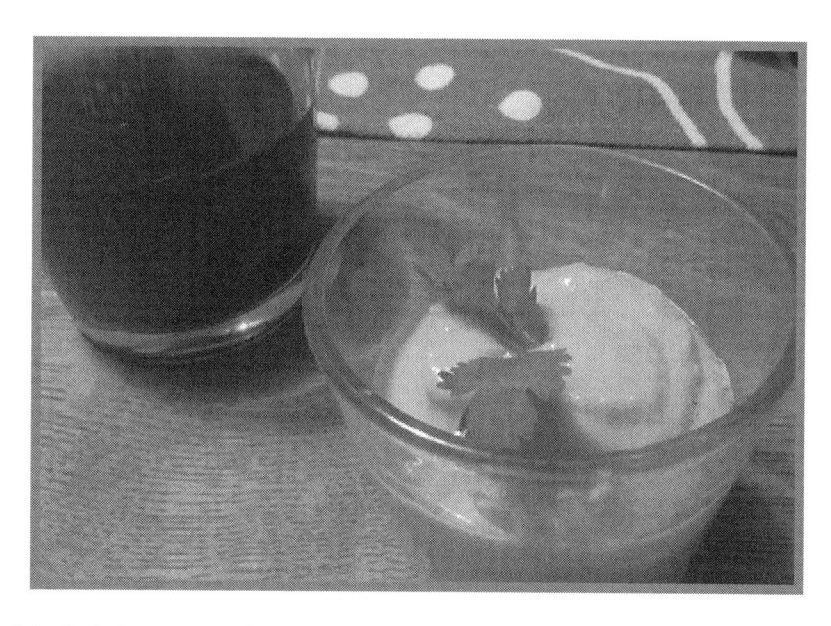

For all of the kale lovers out there, here's the smoothie you've been waiting for! Yes, believe it or not some people actually enjoy the taste of kale, which makes this recipe a deal. While the pineapple juice and fresh fruit will add a bit of sweetness, it won't completely mask the flavor of the kale. This smoothie will give you a sweet, earthy taste while recharging your body with good, natural fuel.

Yields: 2 servings

Ingredients:
1 cup unsweetened almond milk
1 cup packed chopped kale
1/2 cup pineapple juice
1/2 cup diced pineapple
1 banana

Method:
Place all ingredients in blender and blend until smooth.

CHOCOLATE LOVER'S SMOOTHIE

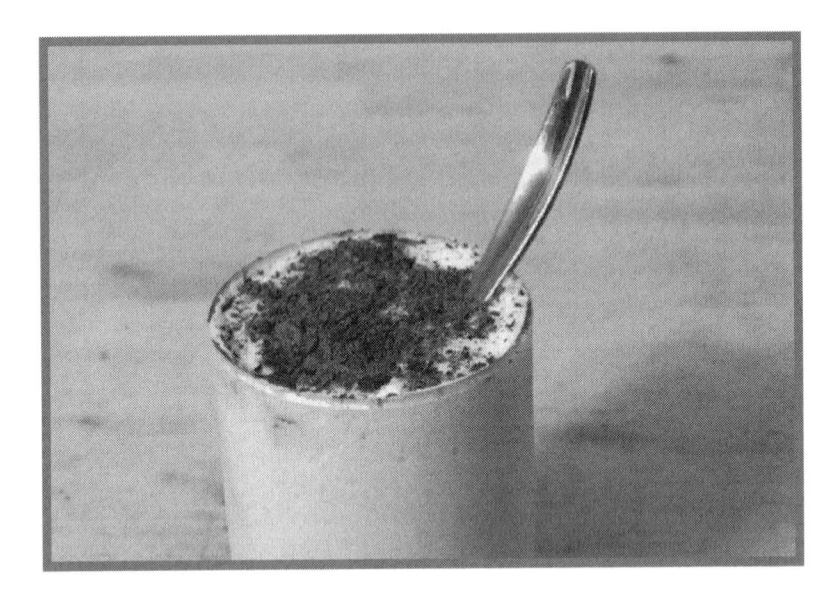

Who says you can't be healthy and have your chocolate, too? This recipe opts for raw cacao powder that can be purchased at a local health food store or online. High in antioxidants, sulfur and magnesium, this is a nutrient rich smoothie that will benefit many areas of your overall health. If it still tastes bitter after adding the dates, feel free to throw in a dash of honey. Also, if you don't like to consume raw eggs, you can omit them from the ingredients without sacrificing too much taste or texture.

Yields: 1 serving

Ingredients:
2/3 cup raw almonds
5 pitted dates
2 frozen bananas, chopped
2 eggs
4 tbsp raw cacao powder
¾ cup water or unsweetened almond milk

Method:
Place all ingredients in blender and blend until smooth.

Printed in Great Britain
by Amazon